A Healing Cancer Handbook

MONIQUE MURPHY

BALBOA.
PRESS

A DIVISION OF HAY HOUSE

Balboa Press books may be ordered through booksellers or by contacting:

Balboa Press
A Division of Hay House
1663 Liberty Drive
Bloomington, IN 47403
www.balboapress.com.au
1 (877) 407-4847

Printed in the United States of America.

ISBN: 978-1-4525-2673-7 (sc)
ISBN: 978-1-4525-2674-4 (e)

Balboa Press rev. date: 01/12/2015

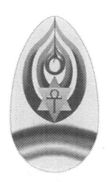

"*My present purpose is not to vaunt a new remedy but to state a fact — that cancer, even when advanced in degree and of long duration, may get better, and does sometimes get well. There is a cure for cancer, apart from operative removal....These cases are the sun of our hope.*" Sir Alfred Pearce Gould

"*Tomorrow, there is always hope & where there is hope, there is life.*"

"*To ensure good health: eat lightly, breathe deeply, live moderately, cultivate cheerfulness and maintain an interest in life.*"
William Londen

Also by Monique Murphy: Self Healing the Body & Beyond

For Marise & Michelle
and all those dealing with cancer

CONTENTS

INTRODUCTION

As my first book *Self Healing The Body & Beyond* came out of my Body Stress Release Practice so this *Healing Cancer Handbook* has come out of my Emotional Freedom Technique Practice.

Working with cancer patients has made me realise there is a real need for succinct, simple information on what they can do to be well once again. I believe we are all responsible for our own health and happiness.

We may need some outside help, but ultimately every healing journey is unique and personal and there is much we can do to aid the process.

The most important thing is to take back your power. Nobody knows what is going on in your body and mind better than you do.

Many of the cancer patients I have worked with are overwhelmed with too many books to read and diets to try, well-meaning friends all have suggestions and ideas to the point where confusion reigns and the sick person stops listening.

This book is a simple attempt to point you in the right direction, a mere guide to finding what might work, for you. It is not suggested that you do all of the protocols but that you search out more information about the ones that appeal to you.

By far the most important factor in healing cancer is a positive mental attitude. You have to believe it is possible. My guess is, you already do; why else would you be reading this book?

The next most important thing is having a health care provider who will listen to you, talk you through all your options and be willing to explore alternatives if you so desire. Anybody who tells you "This is the only way" is not in touch with the latest research. There are many ways to get well and you need to choose the path that most appeals to you. Your belief in a treatment will increase its efficacy.

There is no right or wrong way to deal with cancer; there is only the right way for you.

CHAPTER 1

Common Sense

Integrative medicine is the way of the future, using the best of conventional medicine to treat the existing condition and then using so called "alternative" medicine to ensure an environment in which cancer cannot thrive so that it does not return. Using complementary approaches whilst undergoing conventional treatment will optimise your body's ability to cope with the devastating side effects. Having a health care professional that you really trust is important. To me, that is a doctor who will listen to you, try to find the cause of your illness and eradicate it from that perspective, as opposed to just treating the symptoms.

Personally I am not a fan of surgery, chemotherapy and radiation but sometimes these approaches are necessary. The ideal is to have an oncologist who also specialises in alternative medicine. In this way the ravages of the conventional treatment can be dampened by the anti-oxidative and detoxifying effects of the alternative therapies. If you can't find such an oncologist then at least find one that is open to working within a team of health care specialists that you trust.

All healing is ultimately self-healing. True healing, lasting healing must come from within. The imperatives I recommend are evaluating your diet, cleaning up the chemical environment you live in and examining your emotional health in order to make the necessary change.

Having a strong immune system is essential so that inflammation is reduced and your body can cope with whatever is ailing it. Clearing unresolved emotion issues is an essential part of healing chronic disease as unresolved issues can poison your body physiologically and biochemically. Remember the body and the mind are one entity.

The best way to boost your immune system is to follow an anti-inflammatory (alkalizing) diet, get regular exercise, foster relationships that bring joy and fun into your life, love and accept yourself, let go of any anger, resentment or negative emotions, and reduce environmental toxins wherever possible.

Exercise does not have to be strenuous. Getting some fresh air everyday by walking in nature is excellent as is yoga or even just breathing exercises if you are truly too tired to move around. (See chapter 6 for breathing exercises.)

It will also pay you to remember that genes alone do not determine your health. Only about five to ten per cent of your genes directly determine your health; (Willett 2002) fully ninety per cent of your genes' expression is affected by environmental influences including nutrition, stress and emotions. Dr. Bruce Lipton shows in his book Biology of Belief beyond doubt that the environment of your cells is far more important in determining the health and functioning of your cells. (Reik and Walters2001; Surani 2001) If your mother, grandmother and great-grandmother all died of breast cancer it does not mean you will – unless you hold on to the belief that you will.

Feelings of hopelessness, powerlessness, depression and frustration are often a precursor to chronic illness. The body reacts to early childhood trauma and stress later in life. Unresolved emotional issues have been shown to correlate to diseases that manifest in mid-life if the issues are not resolved. Emotional Freedom Technique is one of the fastest and most effective ways to deal with stress and overwhelming emotions. It is also very helpful for dealing with bad habits and negative thought patterns that may be keeping you ill and stuck. There are several healing EFT exercises in Chapter 8.

There will not be a host of testimonials and personal stories in this book but the list of books and websites at the end will show ample cases where the techniques I write about are proven to work. My previous book *Self Healing the Body & Beyond* has many inspiring personal stories of people who have triumphed over chronic pain and disease. What I have included in this book are some perspectives from other health care providers who have experience with alternative cancer treatments.

CHAPTER 2

Eat right for your type

"Let food be thy medicine and medicine be thy food." Hippocrates

It never ceases to amaze me that the old adage "you are what you eat" is not taken seriously. Your body builds, maintains and repairs your cells with the building materials you provide it. Every person is unique and no one diet will work for all, however, there are some basic, simple rules that do apply to all when it comes to cancer.

CANCER LOVES SUGAR. It thrives in an acid environment. Carbohydrates are sugars.

Cut off its food supply and cancer will not thrive.

Dairy is highly inflammatory so watch the dairy foods.

Generally the rule to apply is eat whole foods, that is, as natural as possible so plenty of raw organic fruit and vegetables. Lots of fiber is good for the gut and acidophilus will help restore gut flora if you have been exposed to antibiotics at any time.

Cut down your meat intake to a small amount every day, that is, not eating meat with every meal. It is often advised to go vegan for a while with cancer and the results speak for themselves. This is a big ask for a lot of people but even if just temporary it will give your body the best chance to detox.

Use good oils like olive, coconut, and flaxseed, and take fish oil supplements if you do not eat oily fish often. Do not use margarine, canola or vegetable oils other than the aforementioned.

Avoid all artificial sweeteners. Instead use stevia or xylitol if you need something to sweeten tea/coffee or baked goods. No processed meat and essentially no processed food at all. Anything in a box on a supermarket shelf is likely to be full of preservatives, additives and sugar, so AVOID it.

Anti-oxidant foods have cancer fighting properties so eat plenty of garlic, ginger, turmeric, basil, rosemary and coriander. Green tea, white tea, essiac and tulsi tea may all help fight the cancer forming free radicals.

Supplements may also help if your diet is not ideal (and let's face it, whose is?) Some suggestions: Vitamins C, D, and A, Selenium, coenzyme Q_{10}, glutathione, resveratrol, and Acidophilus. Please be sure to get professionally prescribed supplements not the off the shelf supermarket ones. Amla, an Ayurvedic plant has wonderful immune-boosting properties. This Indian gooseberry has a huge amount of Vitamin C and, in powder form, is easy to ingest. Melatonin is good for the immune system and will help you sleep, which is critical for healing. Transfer factor supplements can also boost immune function. These are derived from cow colostrum or chicken egg yolk and can be taken as injections or by mouth.

Drink plenty of clean (filtered) water and get regular exercise to get the blood pumping and deep breathing going. The Gerson Protocol (Haught, S.J. Censured for Curing Cancer: The American Experience of Dr. Max Gerson. The Gerson Institute, 1991.) advises regular coffee enemas to help the liver to detox. Making sure your lymphatic system is healthy is also imperative. Lymphatic drainage massage may help or jogging gently on a revitaliser is very beneficial.

Cutting out smoking and drinking alcohol can only help the body in its effort to detox. Take a good look at any environmental toxins you may be exposing yourself to as well. This means checking your insect sprays, deodorant (make sure it is aluminium free), soap, shampoo, washing powder and cosmetics too.

Juicing makes ingesting lots of fruit and vegetables easier but a green smoothie a day is also a good idea as you are not losing the fiber in the food. Essentially you can liquidise any leafy greens with fruit and yogurt and add things like mint or cinnamon to make them palatable. Spirulina, chorella and sea vegetables are also wonderfully nutritious things to add to your daily diet.

A lot of people swear by the diet suggested in Dr. Peter J D'Adamo's book *Eat Right For Your Type*. It is a diet that varies according to your blood type and it does make a lot of sense that individual's dietary requirements will differ according to body chemistry.

As with supplements, the right diet for you will be unique and you may need professional help to find out what foods your body will benefit from the most. Get your blood work done, check your sugar levels and make the necessary dietary changes.

See food list on the next page.

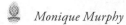

The following list of acid versus alkaline foods will help you make healthy choices:

ACID	ALKALINE
White flour	leafy green vegetables
Sugar	fresh fruit
Grains & cereals	almonds
Fizzy drinks	fresh coconut
Meat	chestnuts
Condiments	acidophilus yogurt/buttermilk
Coffee	herb teas
Alcohol	whey
Dairy products	raw milk
Nuts	kelp
Tinned/preserved fruit	raw honey
Rhubarb	apple cider vinegar
Lentils	avocado
Corn	beets
Beans	mushrooms
Peas	tomatoes

CHAPTER 3

Electromagnetic Stress

"Health means different things to different people. Take time to define what health means to you and what you are willing to do or willing to give up doing to bring better health into your life." Melanie Greenberg Ph.D.

There is growing concern about the link between electromagnetic emissions and cancer. According to articles in The Telegraph in 2012 there have been court rulings where cell phones have been found to cause brain tumours in Europe. (Stephen Adams Medical Corresondent). Excessive or prolonged exposure to electrical, magnetic, wireless or ionizing radiation is not recommended, particularly for children. In his book Anticancer a new way of life, Dr. David Servan-Schreiber recommends that children under twelve should not use cellphones at all. Adults should try to use the 'speaker' function as often as possible or a Bluetooth headset which will reduce the electromagnetic emissions of your mobile phone by a factor of one hundred. He even recommends that you stay away from other people who are using their mobile phones and change ears frequently if on a long call.

This also means trying to avoid living directly under power lines and not using a microwave as well as avoiding x-rays, UV rays and Wi-Fi. Do not carry your cellphone on your body and do not sleep with it next to your bed. Modern technology is wonderful but we must not become totally

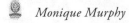

dependent on it and forget the need for balance in our lives. Spending all day in front of a computer screen is not good for anyone but especially not for someone who is already ill.

The same can be said for all day with the radio or television on.

CHAPTER 4

Pray Believing

"Everyone prays in their own language, and there is no language that God does not understand." Duke Ellington

When I say "pray believing" it covers a very large area as prayer is open to interpretation. Defining prayer, like defining "God" is almost impossible. Prayer can be done with or without words, in silence, in gestures and it can even be a subconscious activity rather than a conscious one.

No matter what your religious or spiritual beliefs, I believe prayer/contemplation/meditation needs to form a part of your daily healing protocol. Prayer and intention have been proven to be effective in healing. (Daniel J. Benor, M.D. Complementary Medical Research in 1990)

Why do we have to choose between the rational and the intuitive, the analytical and the spiritual? These are not mutually exclusive. In the same way that you do not have to choose between orthodox and complementary medicine, the one can complement the other.

To me, prayer is not asking for something but it is a quiet state of mindfulness and gratitude for all that is. It is a "tuning in" to the highest and best part of yourself and the Universe. In The Experience of God by Jonathon Robinson Clement of Alexandria described prayer as "conversation" with

God, and I really like that definition. M. Scott Peck describes meditation as listening for God's voice. Perhaps my favourite description is that of Dr. Larry Dossey in his book Healing Words: "Prayer is like that. It is our tie to the Absolute, a reminder of our nonlocal, unbounded nature, of that part of us that is infinite in space and time and is Divine. It is the Universe's affirmation that we are immortal and eternal, that we are not alone."

Being grateful for what you have is the best way to get more of what you want. It is imperative to focus on what you want, not on what you don't want. What you focus on expands and what you think about tends to proliferate. Thoughts really do become things, so if you don't like what is showing up in your life you have to analyse what is going on in both your conscious and your subconscious mind. Beliefs are not right, wrong or even real, they are just thoughts we think over and over until they become entrenched in our mind as beliefs. Subconscious beliefs may also be collected during our formative childhood years; they may not even be ours to begin with. Know that you have the power to change a belief any time you choose to do so. It is very important to take a look at your beliefs and make sure they are serving you.

Your whole life is coloured by your perceptions and your perceptions are based on your beliefs. Particularly if you are sick, you need to look at what limiting beliefs may be in the way of your healing.

What does this mean for the sick person wishing to be well? It means you need to spend more time thinking about wellness than "your illness". It means it is very important to IMAGINE YOURSELF WELL, spend time every day picturing yourself fit and healthy doing all the things you love doing and used to be able to do. You need to have fun playing the "What if" game, and act "as if". Ask yourself: "What if I was well, what would I be doing?"

"What if I was on holiday in Europe, what would that feel like?"

"What if I could be anywhere, doing anything, what would that be?"

Act as if you are well, plan as if you are well, even if you are lying in a hospital bed you can close your eyes and make believe. Pretending is very powerful. This is a game that gets you into the right frame of mind for healing. Visualisation with elevated emotion is the best way to move from where you are to where you want to be.

If you don't already have a "Vision Board" it may be something to start. A "Creation Box" is a similar concept and you can hide it under your bed.

Whether you have a board or a box, the idea is to fill it with images of what you want and look at these every day while feeling how lovely it would be if all these dreams were already true. If you are ill and have been given a diagnosis that suggests you won't be around long, you can buy into it or you can decide that you simply refuse to accept it and plan and dream for your future. Fill your board/box with pictures of you in the future with your children or your grandchildren. Fill your board/box with images of the things you still want to do and places you want to visit. Look at these every day and spend time filling in all the details and FEELING how wonderful it is to experience all these things. Like attracts like so it is very important that you get to a place where you feel fabulous.

The important thing to realise is that your subconscious mind cannot tell the difference between fantasy and reality; if you close your eyes and imagine biting into a lemon your mouth responds as if you really are biting a lemon. Try it for yourself, see? Your mouth filled with saliva didn't it? As far as your subconscious was concerned you really were biting into a lemon! This is the power you have to create a new reality with the thoughts you think, words you speak and expectations you have. Expectation determines outcome.

The key to manifesting what you want in life is to do it in your head first. As George Bernard Shaw said; "Imagination is the beginning of creation. You imagine what you desire, you will what you imagine and at last you create what you will."

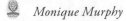

After you spend a few minutes a day doing this creative imagination it is a good idea to give thanks as if it has already happened. Just being grateful for what is good in your life will focus your energy in the right way to bring in more of what you want.

Hippocrates, who lived around 460-377 B.C., stated that: "The natural healing force within each one of us is the greatest force in getting well." There is solid scientific evidence that mind-body techniques do fight disease and foster well-being. There are studies showing that guided imagery can influence the recovery rates for patients with cancer (Dr. Larry Dossey Healing Beyond the Body). Some quiet time is definitely worth adding to your daily "to do" list.

CHAPTER 5

Creative Visualisation

".....our job is first and foremost to simply define the dream, specifically the end result, in every imaginable detail." Mike Dooley

If you want to understand the principles of creative visualisation all you have to remember is that everything is energy. Quantum physics has now proven that nothing is in fact solid; there is space between atoms and sub-atoms. Everything is made up of particles of energy. There is also a field of energy that connects all things in time and space. Energy is magnetic so energy of a certain vibration or quality will attract energy of a similar vibration – like attracts like.

The old saying "as you sow, so shall you reap" is equivalent to saying what you put out, you get back and energetically this is quite true. Essentially this means what you think about, focus on, believe in the most will become true for you. It makes sense then to spend some time every day creating wellness in your mind and body through the practice of guided imagery/creative visualisation.

Creative visualisation: an example

Sit or lie in a comfortable position, close your eyes and breathe deeply, in through the nose and out through the mouth.

Transport yourself to a place of beauty, your special sanctuary – it may be in a forest, on a beach, on a yacht in the middle of the ocean – wherever you can feel truly relaxed.

Picture yourself standing in this place, feel your bare feet on the ground and the warmth of the surface under your feet, feel connected and grounded to the earth. Feel the warmth of the sun on your face or a gentle breeze, smell the flowers or salt air and hear the waves lapping or river burbling beside you.

From the center of the earth feel a warm, golden light coming up through your feet, travelling up your legs and into the base of your spine. As it moves up it feels warm, soothing, healing. From the base of your spine feel the warm, sparkling light travel into your spleen area and radiating out into all the organs, glands and tissues of this area. Next it goes into the solar plexus area, glowing and spinning sending warm, love, and light energy into all the organs, glands and tissues of your mid-section.

After a few more breaths see the golden light travel into your heart; glowing and spinning it gets pumped from your heart into every cell of your body. Every cell in your body is glowing with this sparkling, effervescent energy that heals, soothes and restores as it goes.

Now from above your head, as if coming down from the heavens you see a bright white light energy. This bright white light energy now flows through the top of your head, down into the middle of your forehead and then into your throat. See it travelling slowly down from the top of your head and as it reaches each energy center, see it spinning out to fill the area and heal all the organs, glands and tissues in the area. From the throat you see the white light travel down into your heart where it meets the beautiful golden light that you have drawn up from beneath your feet. The sparkling light energies mix and get pumped out to every cell, organ and tissue of your body, every cell is dancing with joy and rejuvenation. Your whole body feels light and tingling.

See the light energy flowing up from under your feet, through your heart and out of the top of your head and then circling back down the other side, through your heart again and out under your feet – it's as if it is running in a figure 8 or infinity sign all around and through you. If you have any area in particular that is a problem you can spend more time focusing the healing love light energy there. For example, if you have a tumour in your breast then you actively see the energy dissolving the tumour. Or if you have arthritis in your joints then spend a little extra time on the areas that are painful. Otherwise just relax, breathe and picture this healing energy flowing through and around you for 10 to 20 minutes.

If this seems too complex for you, simply relax your entire body and imagine yourself floating in a beautiful warm ocean of water. Then imagine that you are lying on the warm sand and soaking up the nurturing energy of the sun. Focus on just being present in this moment of self-nurturing, let everything else go. Feel grateful and centered and know that all is well in your world. The most important thing is just to feel good and hold on to this feeling for as long as you can. The other thing that can be helpful if you are inclined to listen for your intuition is just quiet your mind, breathe deeply and ask your body what it is trying to tell you? Ask yourself where your life is out of balance and what you might do to restore more balance? Then just listen and see what comes up.

CHAPTER 6

Breathing Exercises

1. Sit or lie in a comfortable position. Take a deep breath in, picture light and energy flowing in with each breath. Every breath you take brings more and more health and well-being into every cell of your body. Hold the breath for a while before exhaling. As you breathe in and out you feel more and more relaxed and calm. The more you breathe and relax the lighter you feel. Picture yourself floating, gently like a cloud in a clear blue sky. Up, up and away you float to wherever you want to be.

2. Making sure you are comfortable, start breathing slowly and deeply, in through the nose and out through the mouth. Start off by picturing red light coming in with each breathe and filling your body. It is a sparkling, shiny, jewel red filling every cell of your body. The red light energises you. Then, breath in a bright, shiny, orange light and send this to all the cells in your body. The orange light you breathe in fills you with strength. Breathe in a bright golden yellow light that fills you with wisdom. Next breathe in a beautiful emerald green which fills you with a feeling of peace, harmony and love. Breathe in love for yourself and love for all around you. Now you breathe in a healing, gentle sky blue light that fills your body and mind with a sense of joy and peace. The next breath is dark, indigo blue and it makes you feel you know beyond your normal sense of knowing.

Breathe in a gentle violet light and feel your spirit soar, relax, breathe gently in and out. See yourself inside a soft pink cloud floating, free, no worries, no cares, no pain just floating free in a pink bubble of unconditional love. Float gently for a while until you want to come softly back to earth feeling refreshed, rejuvenated and relaxed.

3. In this next breathing exercise you are to focus on how you would like to feel. Find a comfortable position and start taking slow, deep breaths in and out. On the in breathe, which should last for the count of between 8 and 12, say silently to yourself "I AM". On the out breathe after holding your breathe for an equal amount of counts say "peace".

Next breathe, breathing in for the count of 8 or 12, say "I AM" hold for the count of 8 to 12 then breathe out saying "calm". Carry on for 10 to 20 minutes with whatever words work for you, for example:

I AM		well
I AM		serene
I AM		relaxed
I AM		whole
I AM		healed
I AM		peace
I AM		love
I AM		light
I AM		joy
I AM		calm
I AM		free
I AM		healthy
I AM		happy
I AM		One with all that is
I AM		all that I AM

Again, continue the exercise for 10 to 20 minutes. You should feel a deep sense of peace and calm after doing this exercise. It may help to light a candle to help you focus or burn some incense.

CHAPTER 7

Love Yourself

What is love? How do we love ourselves and why is it important to do so? Love is caring, nurturing, being kind, tolerant and forgiving. It appears that a great degree of human unhappiness and depression comes from a lack of self-love and self-acceptance.

There seems to be an almost universal lack of self-esteem among the majority of people. Whether this comes from parents who are too busy for us or a school system that too harshly judges and tries to pigeonhole us I cannot say. All I know is that I see it time and again amongst my clients and it makes me extremely sad.

Self-loathing and self-bashing are sure ways to make you sad and sick. Sometimes it is not even a conscious thing but if you listen to your self-speak you may be surprised at how often you berate yourself. So, to be happy and healthy you need to start taking care of yourself, nurturing and being kind to yourself.

This is where you may need a therapist to help you. I advocate an Emotional Freedom Technique Practitioner, Psych-K, hypnotherapy or neuro linguistic programming practitioner (NLP) to help you get your

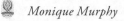

emotional baggage cleared up and your thoughts and words in alignment with a newer, healthier you.

Self-care also means having regular Body Stress Release, massage, reiki, cranio-sacral or osteopathic manipulations. The idea behind this is to keep your spine healthy and your body's communication lines open. Both the autonomic and cerebrospinal nervous systems need to be coordinated and balanced for your body to be healthy.

To love yourself or another means to want the best for them. It means wanting them to be the best they can be, to fully realise their potential. Can we shine that sort of love on ourselves? Are we prepared to completely love and accept ourselves?

CHAPTER 8

EFT

The basic premise of Emotional Freedom Technique is that all negative emotions come from a disruption in the body's energy system. Tapping on the acupressure points, whilst focusing on the problem, breaks the link between the negative thought/feeling/memory and the emotional response. It also restores the body's energy system to balance.

Releasing stored and repressed emotion from the body-mind is imperative for health and healing.

Stress is an exacerbating factor in all illness and EFT is guaranteed to reduce your feelings of stress, fear and anxiety. It may also be used to release physical pain and help you sleep if you are having trouble getting enough rest. Physical pain is often a sign of mental/emotional issues that need examining, suppressing things we don't want to think about is in no way healthy. Getting enough rest is critical to your body's ability to heal and repair itself.

Emotional Freedom Technique diminishes the intensity of emotional trauma and modifies the way the brain processes emotional information. Bearing in mind that your physical body reacts to stress through your breath, your blood pressure and muscle tension affecting your body's ability to function efficiently. Your subconscious runs your body via the autonomic nervous system. The amygdala in the brain has been programmed by childhood experiences that may elicit a flight or fight stress response when something happens later in life that reminds it of the earlier traumatic event. The situation you face may not be a real threat at all but your body will react with a fear response anyway thus lowering your immunity.

Research using brain scans shows that tapping whilst focusing on a problem actually takes the brain out of flight or fight mode and returns it to rest and repair mode. Blood tests before and after tapping show physical changes in the blood proving that actual change is taking place in the body-mind.

The Tapping Points:

Top of the head

Between the eyebrows

Beside each eye

Under the eyes

Under the nose

Under the mouth

Between the collarbones

Under the breasts

Under the arms

Additional tapping points are on the wrist and fingertips.

The Tapping Points

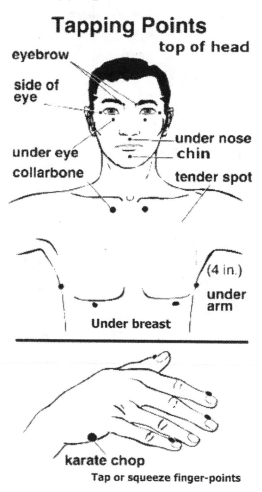

Tapping Points

eyebrow

top of head

side of eye

under nose

chin

under eye

collarbone

tender spot

(4 in.)

under arm

Under breast

karate chop

Tap or squeeze finger-points

1. Tapping points
2. Where and how to tap
3. Psychological Reversal
4. The Set-up Statement
5. The Reminder Phrase
6. Gamut procedure
7. SUD's
8. Putting it all together

Before you begin, ask yourself from 1- 10 how anxious am I feeling about this illness or this diagnosis or this scan or whatever it is you want to focus on? You need to have a "level" in order to measure how the anxiety drops as you go through a few rounds of tapping.

To begin with you tap on the side of the hand, the "karate chop point" and say: "even though I have this diagnosis, I deeply and completely love and accept myself anyway." This is the "set-up statement", do this three times.

Then tap through all the points approximately seven times each spot whilst focusing on the problem/feeling you want to release.

Then, tapping on the top of your head you repeat "this diagnosis"

Tapping between the eyebrows "this diagnosis"

Tapping next to the eyes "this diagnosis"

Tapping under the eyes "this diagnosis"

Tapping under the nose "this diagnosis"

Tapping under the mouth "this diagnosis"

Tapping between the collarbones "this diagnosis"

Tapping under the breasts "this diagnosis"

Tapping under the arms "this diagnosis"

If you want you can then also tap on the wrists and squeeze all your fingertips whilst still focusing on the words "this diagnosis".

Take a deep breath in through the nose and breathe slowly out through the mouth. Tap a few more rounds and focus on whatever you are feeling. Check in and see whether your level of anxiety has dropped?

This basic tapping protocol may be used for anything you are struggling with. The Association for the Advancement of Meridian Energy Techniques is doing ongoing research showing that this simple technique is very powerful for taking you out of "flight or fight" mode in to "rest and repair" mode, which is imperative for healing.

Brain scans show actual changes in the brain during tapping and blood tests done before and after tapping show changes in the blood.

I know it may seem a little odd but believe me, once you start using this tool you will wonder how you ever survived without it!

Instead of repeating the words "this diagnosis" whilst tapping you could substitute:

"This cancer"

"This tumour in my breast"

"This pain in my ..."

"This fear of my scan"

"This fear of death"

"This anger towards…"

"This guilt about…"

"This sadness about…"

"This deep grief about…"

"This fear that the cancer will come back"

"This financial anxiety"

Other common themes to tap on:

"Even though I don't feel good enough"…"I love and accept myself."

"Even though I feel unworthy"

"Even though I feel unlovable"

"Even though I feel nobody cares"

"Even though I feel overwhelmed"

"Even though I did…"

"Even though he did…"

"Even though my mother said…"

"Even though I'm waiting for the test results, I love and accept myself anyway and choose to find peace today."

"Even though I am dying, I love and accept myself anyway and choose to live fully today."

EFT research shows that tapping can reduce physical pain on average by 68% which is pretty encouraging. In other words, we may not be able to reduce the physical cause of the pain but by removing the emotional component you can release two thirds of your pain. Physical pain is often interwoven with emotional pain so by working through all your feelings of anger, fear, frustration, abandonment, self-loathing and lack of self-acceptance you may be surprised by how much healing takes place. Some of my clients have had huge success with things like fibromyalgia and chronic fatigue (both supposedly incurable) simply by releasing unfinished emotional business.

As you tap you may find more and different feelings and memories arising out of your subconscious and this is GREAT. The more you tap the more you may find to tap on but RELEASING all this negative emotion and repressed feeling is the whole point of the exercise.

In Emotional Freedom Technique we sometimes find there are psychological blocks in the way of it working. These are subconscious blocks we may have that are protecting us somehow. The most common ones are:

Is it safe for me to let this go now?

Who will I be if I let this go now?

Am I too angry to let this go now?

Do I deserve to let this go now?

Is it even possible for me to let this go now?

We assume that these may be present and negate them to start off with. If you are tapping on having cancer you may like to include all of these in your "set-up statement" just in case they are blocking the effectiveness of the tapping. For example, your set-up may be:

"Even though I have this cancer, I deeply and completely love and accept myself anyway" (repeated three times)

"Is it safe for me to be well now? Who will I be without this cancer? Am I too angry to let this cancer go now? Do I even deserve to be well? I have this cancer in my body and I wonder if it is possible that it could go away?" You say all of these whilst tapping on the various acupressure points as per the diagram.

Then tapping through all the points from the top of the head down just keep asking yourself what else is possible? Then you move on to actually affirming that yes, it is possible.

Whilst tapping through all the points you might affirm:

"I believe it is safe for me to let this cancer go now"

"I believe I will know who I am when I am cancer free"

"I am not too angry with myself or anyone else to let this cancer go now"

"I know I deserve to be well"

"I absolutely believe it is possible for me to let this cancer go now"

One of my favourite types of tapping is "Temporal Tapping". This is tapping around the ears, on the temporal lobe to change negative limiting beliefs and or bad habits. This tapping needs to be done every day, preferably twice a day on ONE belief/habit until it has shifted, only then do you move on to another one.

Tap in a circular motion, from the front of the ear around towards the back and bottom of the ear (on the LEFT of the head to tap out the negative and on the RIGHT side to tap in the positive). We use 6 different pronouns because we are not sure where the belief is held in the subconscious mind and we want to clear it all out.

If you have been told you have only two years to live for example and you want to shift this belief you would tap each of the following three times around the left ear saying:

"I no longer need to believe I have only 2 years to live"

"You no longer need to believe you have only 2 years to live"

"She/he no longer needs to believe she/he has only 2 years to live"

"*Name* no longer needs to believe *Name* has only 2 years to live"

(Put your name in the above sentence)

"We no longer need to believe we have only 2 years to live"

"They no longer need to believe they have only 2 years to live"

Take a deep breath in and breathe out slowly then start tapping in the positive around the right ear three times each:

"I would really like to believe I have a long and healthy life ahead"

"You would really like to believe you have a long and healthy life ahead"

"She/he would really like to believe she/he has a long and healthy life ahead"

"*Your Name* would really like to believe *your Name* has a long and healthy life ahead"

"We would really like to believe we have a long and healthy life ahead"

"They would really like to believe they have a long and healthy life ahead"

Deep breathe in and slowly out again. What you are doing with this temporal tapping is creating new neural pathways in your brain so habitual negative thoughts are changed to more healthy and constructive ones.

It can be successfully used for weight loss, stopping smoking, changing emotional eating patterns and much more.

You have about 60,000 thoughts every day and a full 54,000 are below your conscious awareness. Most often you repeat the same thoughts every day. Surely it makes sense to pay attention to what you are thinking and feeling? If thoughts become things, and they do, it is time to take control of this very powerful force within you.

If this is too hard alone then find an EFT Practitioner to help you. Having even just a few sessions with a professional will help you to understand the process and apply it more effectively to any aspect of your life that needs healing.

Clinical Psychologist Patricia Carrington Ph.D. developed what is known as the EFT Choices Protocol which I have found particularly useful both personally and with clients. With the Choices method we change the set-up and reminder phrases to suit the exact situation we find ourselves in.

For example, instead of saying: "even though I am afraid the cancer may come back, I deeply and completely love and accept myself anyway" we would say: "even though I am afraid the cancer may come back, I choose to believe I am and will remain cancer free."

So to come up with an effective "choice", we need to look at what is and change it to what we would like instead. Some more examples:

Even though I feel sad when I think of my dad, I choose to feel calm and relaxed when I think of my dad.

Even though I feel frustrated about my lack of success, I choose to feel peaceful and accepting of where I am.

Even though I find it hard to speak in public, I choose to let it be easy and fun to speak to a crowd.

Even though I never felt loved by my parents, I choose to believe my parents loved me very much.

Even though I feel ignored by my husband, I choose to believe my presence and opinions are valuable.

Even though I feel fat, I choose to love my body and see it improving every day.

Get the picture?

Whilst tapping on the karate chop point (the fleshy side of the hand) we repeat our set-up statement and reminder phrase three times, that is:

"Even though I have been ill, I choose to let it be easy to create health every day."

Then we tap through all the points from the top of the head down repeating the first part.

"Even though I have been ill" tap, tap, tap on the head

"Even though I have been ill" tap, tap, tap above the eyes

"Even though I have been ill" tap, tap, tap next to the eyes

"Even though I have been ill" tap, tap, tap below the eyes

"Even though I have been ill" tap, tap, tap beneath the nose

"Even though I have been ill" tap, tap, tap below the mouth

"Even though I have been ill" tap, tap, tap on the collarbone

"Even though I have been ill" tap, tap, tap beneath the breasts

"Even though I have been ill" tap, tap, tap under the arms

Then we start again at the top of the head repeating the second part, our positive choice, tap through all the points whilst saying: "I choose to let it be easy to create health every day."

The third and final round of tapping through all the points we alternate the first and the second part of our statement: "even though I have been ill" tapping on the top of the head then" I choose to let it be easy to create health every day" tapping above the eyes. "Have been ill" tapping next to the eyes; "choose to let it be easy to create health," tapping below the eyes; "have been ill," tapping below the nose; "choose to let it be easy to create health," tapping below the mouth etc. It does not matter at which acupressure point you finish as long as you always end with your positive affirmation, the outcome you choose to create. This applies to all tapping always, it doesn't matter if you miss a point just carry on and don't get hung up on the words you are saying, just focus on the feelings and let the tapping do the work.

One of the most important things to remember when using Emotional Freedom Technique, that is, tapping, is to be specific. Focus on one specific memory or event at a time do not tap generally or globally as this is not likely to bring fast, effective relief. Very often a problem has arisen over time from a number of different happenings, so tapping on "low self-esteem" for example would not be as effective as tapping on the memory of specific events that led you to develop the low self-esteem. For example: "even though my dad scolded me" and "even though my teacher yelled at me" and "even though my first boyfriend left me for my best friend." It is often very helpful to think back to the first time you remember feeling a certain way as much emotion may be buried as a result of one traumatic event at an impressionable age.

CHAPTER 9

Homeopathy for cancer

By Rosemaree Mathers Dip. Hom. RC
Hom. Classical Homeopath

Homeopathy seeks to stimulate the body's own capacity for self-healing and renewal.

As any good homeopath will tell you, homeopathy cannot cure cancer. But what it is capable of doing is to help alleviate some of the stress and trauma of cancer and particularly some of the side effects of radiation and chemotherapy treatment. It can also be extremely beneficial around the huge fears associated with the disease. Homeopathy can be used alongside conventional treatment.

Homeopathy has been practised for over two hundred years.

Its therapeutic principles are very different from those of conventional medicine, as is its concept of ill health and the approach to patients. The homeopathic premise is that disease is not a set of symptoms, but an underlying disturbance of a person's 'vital force'.

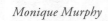

Homeopathic treatment will seek to stimulate the body's own capacity to self-healing and repair. It treats using the principle of "like treats like" and prescribes the medicine that will produce similar symptoms in a healthy person.

A Homeopath taking the initial consultation will take all the physical symptoms and history, but will also ask about your mental and emotional state of mind. A homeopathic consult can expect to take up to an hour and a half.

The remedy that is prescribed is specific to your personality, constitution and lifestyle. Often the consultation in itself is therapeutic.

Commonly asked questions

How safe is Homeopathy?
    A. It is one of the safest systems of treatment available. If the incorrect remedy is given, it will do no harm. Curative reactions to a remedy may sometimes occur, that is, a profuse sweat, streaming nose, bout of diarrhea, but such happenings (called aggravations) are eliminations and therefore benefit the system which is ready to get rid of what is toxic or harmful.

How do homeopathic remedies differ from orthodox medicine?
    A. Homeopathy belongs to physics while allopathy (conventional medicine) belongs to chemistry. Homeopathy is the application of so-called 'energy medicine' while allopathy depends on chemicals. The tiny white pills or liquid are carriers of dynamic energy and act like radio waves to resonate with the individual's symptoms.

How is homeopathy complementary to allopathy if it is alternative?
    A. Sometimes patients who have been taking a lot of drugs will look for another option to avoid putting further chemicals into their already overloaded system.

The homeopathic medicine does not interfere with the necessary effects of the drugs and the proprietary drugs do not necessarily prevent the remedies from working.

What are remedies made from?

A. Animal, vegetable, mineral. A remedy is made because someone has recognised inherent and latent dynamic energy that is peculiarly characteristic of the raw material substance, for example, Apis mellifera - the bee - is beneficial in that its stings cause the parts to become hot and swollen. Remedies are made in homeopathic pharmacies.

Why should I use homeopathy?

A. Homeopathy is safe, gentle, effective and extremely cost effective. Homeopathy has stood the test of time and is well used in many parts of the world. Many highly respected homeopaths have spent their lives studying and researching the use of homeopathy in the treatment of cancer (for example, Dr. A.U. Ramakrishnan and Catherine R Coulter). Research continues around the world amongst the homeopathic community with many positive results.

CHAPTER 10

A Herbalist's View

By Malcolm K. Harker MHD
Medical Herbalist, Waipu, New Zealand

The last thing that I thought I would ever get was cancer. I used to spell cancer with a capital 'C', but since seeing how easy it is to deal with, in my case at least, I now spell the word with a lower case 'c', to show the contempt I feel for their appearance. On the other hand, I am grateful for their appearance as otherwise how would I learn about them intimately?

My first tumour in 2007 rose to the height of almost 20 millimetres upon my right shoulder, with a width of nearly 30 millimetres, over a three year period whilst I hit it with everything I had available to me. After three years the growth had slowed down and was now floating on top of my skin and could be wobbled from side to side, but it would not fall off. Fed up with the darn thing, I had it scalped off and the surgeon was surprised how clean and pus-free the base was. Pleased to be free at last from my unwelcome friend, it wasn't about to leave me that easily, and for the next three years I had to deal with metastasized baby tumours that came up every seven or eight months or so. However, I was expecting these as I had allowed the first big growth to be surgically removed because I was impatient to see the end of it.

Fearing that I would be inundated with these things soon, I began drinking two litres of spinach and carrot juice daily, fasted off and on for several weeks, two or three days at a time, drinking ultra violet light-treated rain water only, and supped three times daily a cup of strong warm tea of fresh chickweed. When I couldn't find enough chickweed I used dried chickweed, often available in health shops such as 'Puti Puti Ra Organics' in Walton Street, Whangarei. Chickweed has potency over several forms of cancers.

I enjoyed being tumor-free for about two or three years after that then they began again, first as an irritation that needs scratching often. This irate spot soon developed a pin head-size spot like a pimple, but it did not go away. Instead it persisted for weeks, sometimes months, continually itching. Eventually it begins to grow bigger and when left will attain a size that becomes harder to deal with. I do not let them get that far - nowhere near.

My immediate strategy is to dab the juice of the Greater Celandine herb (Chelidonium majus) straight onto the 'pimples', whereupon after several applications the little beasties blacken and shrivel away to a hard, crusty scab that soon falls off leaving good, pink, healthy skin beneath.

I had about twenty of these cheeky growths come up, and each succumbed to the yellow juice. However, this is only effective in the mid-summer time when the juice of the plant is at its most potent and with a deep yellow ochre color. In winter, the juice, or sap, is not as strong and has no escharotic (tumor-dissolving) effect. The white latex-like sap of the small Euphorbia herbs (E. helioscopia and E. peplus) that grow so plentifully here in Northland is also escharotic but not, at least in my experience, as active as Celandine. Summer Dandelion juice can also be used with some success over early growths, though the most potent over older warts and growths is definitely the midsummer sap of Celandine.

During the 1970's I suffered dreadful bowel extension problems which my doctor told me may be the sign of early colon and bowel cancer. They found multiple diverticulosis throughout the lower colon and bowel for which drugs were given to no avail. Surgery seemed to be the only option;

so I was told. I didn't believe them and began fasting seriously but could only manage up to two weeks without craving food. I made fresh carrot, celery and spinach juices every morning and ate only raw fresh vegetables, especially the brassica family of mustard, broccoli, cabbage and kale, every morning for breakfast and every other meal of the day with a little cooked food to break the monotony, such as fried onions, mushrooms, beans and white soft sheep's cheese, very occasionally, but no meat at this time.

After three months on fresh carrot and home-made grape juices, plus loads of fresh, raw salads, I awoke one morning in shock to see I was leaking lumpy, dark pus-like matter from the bladder. Initial shock turned to great joy when I realised that what I was going through was an elimination of the cancerous matters, and slowly my energies, skin color and confidence returned. I was detoxing due to my own efforts, and that felt good. Adult nappies were resorted to catch the eliminations over the next couple of months or so. I have had no such intestinal-bowel trouble since and that was in the mid 1970's

During the 2000's, the baking soda and maple syrup cancer remedy became popular and several people who tried the recipe reported that they were now in remission from cancer and a couple whom I gave the treatment recipe to have reported that they have been clear for over two or three years, even though they were originally given only a few months to live by their doctor. The website for this recipe is www.cancertutor.com/kelmun/ One lady wrote to me recently telling me that she was supposed to be dead two years ago according to her doctor, except she takes this remedy often to keep it at bay. Diatomaceous earth has anti-carcinogenic properties and we take this every day with a probiotic drink because this natural silica-rich powder from ancient deep sea beds is reputed to scrape away the coating of harmful bacteria, parasites and viruses, as well as cancerous cells.

For more information go to www.denz.co.nz

Cannabis. One of the world's most positive anti-cancer treatments is from a banned herb in this country, though Cannabis is fast earning a much deserved good reputation medicinally – at last. Traditional herbalists will one day be legally entitled to use this herb in its pure oil form to rid the body of all cancers within a few months. For more information go to <u>www.cureyourowncancer.org/rick-simpson.html</u> Unable to use this great herb for a recent fast growing tumor, I made up a paste using old Bloodroot powder, Golden Seal root powder, Cayenne and car battery acid (sulphuric acid), which I knew had just the right degree of acidity not to burn a hole through my body. Whilst this may sound like a hairy mountain man's way to heal, the fact is that sulphuric acid whether from a car battery or from a pharmaceutical company is identical in action, and eats gently into the tumor whilst taking down the escharotic herb powders with it, with minimal irritation. The end result can be seen in the accompanying photos. Whilst I would not recommend this rather graphic way to deal with a so-called incurable disorder, one can purchase various escharotic creams and pastes that are reputed to do the same job, though one I tried called 'Black salve' was almost impossible to bear on the growth site, so powerfully painful and stinging it was on the skin.

I also used an IFAS violet ray unit to help destroy each tumor. I gave the growths six minutes exposure every morning, before putting the Celandine juice or the Golden seal salve on them. Mostly they shrink and disappear within six or seven weeks.

This has been my personal experience in cancer remission.

Please note that I do not and cannot supply the above mentioned ingredients or products.

Sincerely,
Malcolm K. Harker MHD. Waipu.

CHAPTER 11

A Naturopath's Approach

By Karen Creighton MH, Iridologist, BET

As a natural health practitioner with over 25 years of working in the industry (my early years working in the UK specialising in incurable diseases) I have found that there is definitely no one programme fits all.

After a few years of having my own practice, I started working with clients who were dealing with "incurable illnesses". I worked with a specific programme which included raw foods only and most of the food intake was in the form of juices and superfoods, with herbals to help support all of the detoxification pathways. This programme worked wonderfully well with some, bringing about a complete turnaround in their lives, but didn't bring any results with others.

This sent me on a voyage of discovery which continues today; I went on to study, bioenergy medicine. This helped me to use machines that can ascertain what is going on energetically in an individual's body. The modern ones we use today can also help us to find the optimum way of bringing about balance and enable the system to heal itself.

After these years of study and experience, I treat each client individually. I feel this is the best way to go. When a client comes to me, no matter what we are dealing with, I ask them what their symptoms are. They obviously tell me why they are here, so we know that they have a diagnosis. I do take this into account but it is not what I focus on. I put an emphasis on how and what they are feeling, past health history, their eating habits and their environment. All of which are important for us to get a complete picture.

We then put them on to our energy scan to see where there are energy blockages, I then go on to find remedies that will help unblock them. It is interesting that with the Etascan – our scanning device – although the cancer might be in the breast or pancreas, the blockage is normally in another area of the body like the liver or stomach, or anywhere else for that matter!

What I have found fascinating working with these bio-energy devices is that we find many different pathogens that have been lurking for what could be decades within the body causing a lowering of a person's whole system, by lowering the body's vital energy, then tumours can develop – as an example.

Linda – Linda came to see us 5 years ago and she had a diagnosis of breast cancer. Linda had decided that she wasn't going to go down the medical route. This decision was made without any consultation with any practitioner. After having therapy with another practitioner working on the emotional side, she came to me at the clinic and we went over her health history. A few things jumped out at me – one was glandular fever, Linda had Glandular fever as a teenager very badly. The other was she had reacted to her BCG vaccination a few years prior to that. She was also very sensitive to many foods and so her diet was quite limited.

The scan showed up some very interesting things – Linda was affected by not only the glandular fever virus (Epstein Barr) she had 5 others lurking within her cells. Most of this showed up in her liver and digestive tract. In my experience when you have a viral overload like this nearly everyone has food intolerances.

By finding these things out it enabled us to put Linda onto a programme designed to help kill off or reduce the viral overload, and bring her energy up. I put an emphasis on making sure that the body has the right building blocks to make healthy cells. The most important (in my opinion) nutrients are our minerals. I make sure that everyone is supplementing with at least Magnesium and some of the others along with lots of healthy vegetables, fats and proteins. With Linda I got her on Magnesium oil, which she put on her skin (it absorbs really well that way), selenium and Himalayan black salt to cover all the trace minerals plus sulphur.

By using these strategies she enabled her body to heal itself including the cancer.

In Linda's words...

"After going on the scan Karen put me onto a specific diet which took into account my own personal preferences and needs, this was actually very easy to follow, and some homeopathic and nutritional supplements. Plus she recommended that I visit another practitioner that could help me with some relaxation techniques.

After 6 months of visiting Karen every month to check that all was going well, I started to feel an energy level that I hadn't experienced for a very long time. I felt a lot of subtle shifts in me that were hard to explain but I knew I was getting better. I went back to my oncologist and had some scans and I was given the all clear, they couldn't believe it, but I could. I knew my body was feeling so good, it had to be well, I had check-ups every 6 months for the past few years and I have now finally been given the all clear.

The cancer scare has been such a gift. If I hadn't had the diagnosis I would never have taken stock of my life and made the changes I have plus I have never felt this good and so for that I am so very grateful."

In the last year or so I have been doing research and working on a preventative programme which is aimed at boosting the body's ability to heal itself. By working to remove pathogens (viruses, bacteria, fungus and parasites) we bring about a breeding ground for good health and on top of that we make sure that there is optimum nutrition for the individual to enable energy to flow freely and abundantly. This is what we work on at Reviresco – optimum health for the individual.

I am blessed to be doing the work that I do and know that I am a cog in a wheel that helps many to achieve their health goals. Whether it is to achieve balanced hormones, to lose weight, sort out digestion, or to make some radical shifts so that people can get over a dis-ease process that many consider incurable.

CHAPTER 12

A Personal & Professional Perspective

By Dr. Mike Louw MB ChB.F.C. Psych (SA)

"Nothing ever goes away until it has taught us what we need to know."
Pema Chodron

The first time the word cancer came up in my life was in my mid-teens. I found out some months later that my mother had undergone a "super radical mastectomy" while I was away at boarding school. Seven years later when I was a medical student my mother spent a few months getting chemotherapy at the same hospital that I was being trained at. This gave me the opportunity to visit her twice a day and do what I could to make her comfortable. At the time I made a promise to myself that I would not feel any guilt when she passed. Instead I would visit daily and do everything I could for her.

Another part of my approach was to seek out spiritual resources to help with my understanding of and coping with death. Particularly powerful was reading Eastern philosophies which I could relate to immediately despite my Christian upbringing, the message of which I took on board instantly. She experienced some uncomfortable side effects from the chemo she went through. The candida infection she had for 6 weeks before it was

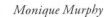

diagnosed was particularly distressing for me to helplessly witness as a medical student.

During the last year of her life her focus on life changed significantly. My mother had been very concerned about her image and status and how we compared to other families materially. In that last year this all changed. She became involved in an inter-racial group "Women for Peace" and helped organise initiatives for the underprivileged non-white children living in our city.

I remember reading her a verse from a Peruvian folk song:

I grow a white rose by Jose Marti

I grow a white rose,
For the true friend
Who gives me his hand freely
For him who wills me ill and tires
This heart with which I live,
Neither thistles nor nettles I grow:
I grow the white rose.

Immediately on hearing this she asked me to get her a copy. I thought at the time something "big" had happened to her on a spiritual level. By spiritual I mean that which pertains to meaning and purpose in life.

Shortly after she passed on my father came into my room at 3 a.m. to say the hospital had just phoned the news. I couldn't tell him that she had spoken to me just before this to tell me she was happy and was where she needed to be. Fortunately I was able to accept the fact and time of her passing and can honestly say I was never troubled by grief. In part this was because I remembered how much pain she had to endure in the last few months of her life.

These experiences may have helped me spiritually but seriously impacted in a negative way on my attitude to modern medical treatment. Did we have to approach medical treatment as a battle, a war we had to win?

I noticed that in my mother's case spiritual growth took place in the context of a terminal illness. Medical research has demonstrated that many factors may contribute to illnesses such as cancer. These factors include smoking, alcohol use, diet, exposure to radiation and other environmental toxins.

Psychological factors on their own are viewed as a weak causative factor according to the U.S. National Cancer Institute.

Depression and anxiety can however significantly impact on quality of life for people with cancer and their caregivers. As a psychiatrist our focus is on diagnosing and treating mental disorders of which depression and anxiety are common in this context. We can do many things to reduce distress but not a lot to aid healing. The word "psychiatry" though is derived from the Greek "psyche" meaning "mind or soul" and "-iatry" meaning "treatment or healing". Relief can come from medication. From psychotherapy and spiritual practices there is greater chance of some form of healing as well as stress reduction taking place.

Healing can occur on one or more levels: mind, spirit and body. There is a good deal of research evidence that spirituality enhances resilience to both serious physical illness and depression. So when faced with a life threatening illness we may consider the possible benefits of adding a spiritual approach to our other coping strategies.

Much later in life I began to reflect on the possibility that a diagnosis of cancer, which is often associated with a threat to life, also by its nature, brought spiritual questions to the fore. Why are we here and what are we supposed to do? When time seems limited and we are suffering these questions become more prominent. Could "cancer" sometimes be a messenger telling us that our life direction is majorly out of balance? If we got the message would the messenger still be necessary? Certainly some

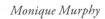

people would cope better with their illness and a few may even recover by going down this path.

Unfortunately there are no guarantees that any one treatment or approach will work for everybody. Building resilience though will make a difference to the quality of life of the person with cancer and to their family and caregivers.

As a psychiatrist I would recommend exploring psychological resilience, spiritual resilience and using social supports as well as treating any depressive illness or anxiety.

"The Road to Resilience" is a psychological approach from the American Psychological Association website (see http://www.apa.org/helpcenter/road-resilience.aspx).

Spiritual resilience is undoubtedly important. See the National Cancer Institute "Relation of Religion and Spirituality to Adjustment, Quality of Life, and Health Indices." See: http://www.cancer.gov/cancertopics/pdq/supportivecare/spirituality/HealthProfessional/page3

What form this takes will need to be a personal choice depending on each individual's beliefs and their philosophy of life. The article notes a negative correlation between the existential well-being scores and anxiety and depression scores.

Social support has been shown by research to extend survival. For example, a study of a million patients published in 2013 confirmed that married patients were diagnosed earlier, stuck with treatment and survived longer than their single counterparts. "Marital Status and Survival in Patients With Cancer," in *Journal of Clinical Oncology* JCO.2013.49.6489.

CHAPTER 13

Death is Inevitable

"When you have a potentially terminal disease, it concentrates the mind wonderfully. It gives a new intensity to life. You discover how many things you have taken for granted – the love of your spouse, the Beethoven symphony, the dew on the rose, the laughter on the face of your grandchild." Archbishop Desmond Tutu

If we know for certain we are going to die, as we all do, how is it that we do not prepare for the inevitable? Every single person on the face of the earth is going to die and not one of us actually knows when our time is likely to be up. We are in fact all in the process of dying right now, one day at a time.

When facing death and dis-ease we need to look at more than just the physical. Dying is a process that involves body, mind and spirit. It behooves us then to think about the end of our lives whether we are sick or well, young or old. We need to ask ourselves, if I were in fact terminally ill with a finite period left to live, would I live differently? In preparing to die, we fully embrace life. Living and dying well both involve some introspection, thinking about your sense of who you are and what you are about. We need to inspect our relationship with ourselves and with others.

Seek forgiveness, again examining anything you may have done to hurt yourself as well as others. What does it mean to forgive someone? It means letting go of any anger, resentment, blame or desire for revenge. It does not mean condoning what someone did or forgetting how a person has wronged you. You do not have to excuse or forget the wrong done to you but you do have to release the negative emotions surrounding it. Forgiveness is good for your health and your peace of mind; it may make no difference to the person who has harmed you but it will make a big difference to your state of mind. It is never too late to make amends, even if someone who has wronged you (or someone you have wronged) is no longer on earth, you can still do the necessary forgiveness work and find peace as a result. No words need be spoken; you can do this work silently or write it all down and burn it. It doesn't matter, as long as you get it off your chest. A written life review can be a very therapeutic tool. If you are not able then ask someone to do it for you, just relate your life story to them and get them to write it down.

Be honest, admit your mistakes, take responsibility for your decisions and actions and let it all go. Often taking stock helps us resolve issues and reconcile internal conflicts we haven't had the courage to face.

Know that you did the best you could with what you had available at the time, we all make mistakes, have regrets, but life is for learning and perhaps teaching.

Suffering is part of life. Some have physical pain, others suffer very real psychological and emotional pain. In truth I don't think you can separate them. According to Nietzsche, suffering ends when we find meaning and purpose in it. Possibly the hardest thing is to watch someone you love suffering, however for the sick or dying person it is paramount that you do. Just bear witness to the person's pain and suffering. Listen to them, really hear what they are saying for, as hard as it may be, you are doing them a great service. Just being with them, even if a person is not conscious, your presence is purposeful.

Lastly and perhaps most importantly, we need to examine our relationship with the Divine, the spiritual or transcendent part of ourselves and our world. Make peace with your Creator however you conceive Him or Her to be. There is nothing that is unforgiveable in this life, people make mistakes, miss the mark, but that is part of being human. Confronting the inevitability of death frees us to enjoy life. It also encourages us to find meaning in life, to create a life of meaning. If you have any fear that death is the end I encourage you to read about near death experiences and reincarnation. Meditate to try and reach the infinite, transcendent part of your being, there can be nothing more reassuring than this. If you have questions the doctors can't answer, talk to theologians and philosophers until you are satisfied. Always plan for the future, release the past and enjoy the present moment.

I wish you everything of the very best on your journey.

RESOURCES AND RECOMMENDED READING

www.emofree.com

www.eftuniverse.com

www.thewellnesswarrior.com.au

www.gerson.org

www.kriscarr.com

www.dr-gonzalez.com

www.oasisofhope.com

www.connealymd.com

www.cancerresearchsecrets.com

www.healinginsideout.co.nz

www.deepliving.com

The Gerson Miracle, Dying to have known. www.gerson.org. Film, Steve Kroschel

The Beautiful Truth. Film 2008. www.gersonmedia.com

Cancer is Curable. Film 2011. www.programs.naturalnews.com

The Tapping Solution. Nick Ortner. Hay House Inc. 2013. thetappingsolution. com

Ask and it is Given. Esther and Gerry Hicks. Hay House Inc. 2004

A Time To Heal. Beata Bishop. First Stone Publishing 2005. www. canceractive.com

Anticancer a new way of life. Dr. David Servan-Schreiber. Penguin Books 2008. www.anticancerbook.com

Beyond the Relaxation Response. Dr. Herbert Benson. Times Books 1984. www.beyondtherelaxationresponse.org

Cancer: A Nutritional/Biochemical Approach. Henry Osiecki. Bioconcepts Publishing 2002. www.trove.nla.gov.au/work/8489204

Crazy Sexy Diet. Kris Carr. Morris Book Publishing 2011. www.kriscarr.com

Creative Imagery for Meditation. Spectrum SOHL Publications 1989

Creative Visualization. Shakti Gawain. Bantam Books 1979

Eat Right for your Type. Dr. Peter J. D'Adamo. Penguin Putman Inc. 1996. www.dadamo.com

Healing Cancer World Summit. Kevin Gianni. www.renegadehealth.com

Healing the Gerson Way. Charlotte Gerson. Totality Books 2007

Healing Words. Larry Dossey M.D. Harper Collins 1993

Mind over Medicine. Lissa Rankin M.D. Hay House 2013. wwwlissarankin.com

Infinite Possibilities. Mike Dooley. Atria Books 2009. www.tut.com

Molecules of Emotion. Candace B. Pert Ph.D. Touchstone 1999. www.candacepert.com

Sick and Tired. Dr. Robert O. Young. Woodland Publishing 2001. www.phmiracleliving.com

The Edgar Cayce Remedies. William McGarey M.D. Bantam Books 1983

The EFT Manual. Dawson Church. Energy Psychology Press 2013. www.eftuniverse.com

The God Experience. Jonathon Robinson. Hay House 1994

You Can Conquer Cancer. Ian Gawler. Michelle Anderson Publishing 1984. www.gawler.org

ABOUT THE AUTHOR

Monique lives on the edge of the Whangarei Harbour in beautiful Northland, New Zealand with her Kiwi husband.

Passionate about the body's innate ability to restore and heal itself this is Monique's second book on the subject.

Having grown up mainly in South Africa with some years spent in England and Holland, Monique now calls New Zealand home.

Her hobbies include cooking, gardening, walking and boating with her ex-Navy husband. Frequent return visits to family in South Africa keep Monique busy when she is not teaching Emotional Freedom Technique at her regular Workshops.